Electrocardiogram
for
Undergraduate Students

Electrocardiogram
for
Undergraduate Students

Amar R Pazare
MBBS, MD (Medicine)

Professor and Head
Department of Medicine
Seth GS Medical College and KEM Hospital
Mumbai

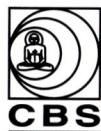

CBS

CBS Publishers & Distributors Pvt Ltd

New Delhi • Bengaluru • Chennai • Kochi • Kolkata • Mumbai
Hyderabad • Jharkhand • Nagpur • Patna • Pune • Uttarakhand

ELECTROCARDIOGRAM
for
Undergraduate Students

ISBN: 978-93-87085-21-3

Copyright © Author and Publisher

First Edition: 2018

Published by Satish Kumar Jain and Produced by Varun Jain for

CBS Publishers & Distributors Pvt Ltd

4819/XI Prahlad Street, 24 Ansari Road, Daryaganj, New Delhi 110 002, India.
Ph: 23289259, 23266861, 23266867   Fax: 011-23243014   Website: www.cbspd.com
e-mail: delhi@cbspd.com; cbspubs@airtelmail.in.
Corporate Office: 204 FIE, Industrial Area, Patparganj, Delhi 110 092
Ph: 4934 4934   Fax: 4934 4935   e-mail: publishing@cbspd.com; publicity@cbspd.com

Branches

- **Bengaluru:** Seema House 2975, 17th Cross, K.R. Road,
  Banasankari 2nd Stage, Bengaluru 560 070, Karnataka
  Ph: +91-80-26771678/79   Fax: +91-80-26771680   e-mail: bangalore@cbspd.com
- **Chennai:** 7, Subbaraya Street, Shenoy Nagar, Chennai 600 030, Tamil Nadu
  Ph: +91-44-26680620, 26681266   Fax: +91-44-42032115   e-mail: chennai@cbspd.com
- **Kochi:** Ashana House, No. 39/1904, AM Thomas Road, Valanjambalam,
  Ernakulam 682 016, Kochi, Kerala
  Ph: +91-484-4059061-65   Fax: +91-484-4059065   e-mail: kochi@cbspd.com
- **Kolkata:** 6/B, Ground Floor, Rameswar Shaw Road, Kolkata-700 014, West Bengal
  Ph: +91-33-22891126, 22891127, 22891128   e-mail: kolkata@cbspd.com
- **Mumbai:** 83-C, Dr E Moses Road, Worli, Mumbai-400018, Maharashtra
  Ph: +91-22-24902340/41   Fax: +91-22-24902342   e-mail: mumbai@cbspd.com

Representatives

- **Hyderabad** 0-9885175004
- **Jharkhand** 0-9811541605
- **Nagpur** 0-9021734563
- **Patna** 0-9334159340
- **Pune** 0-9623451994
- **Uttarakhand** 0-9716462459

Printed at Rashtriya Printers, Delhi, India

Foreword

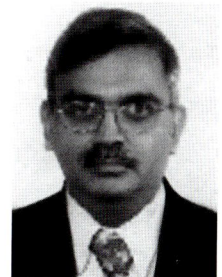

It gives me immense pleasure to write the Foreword to this book *Electrocardiogram for Undergraduate Students* written by Dr Amar R Pazare, Professor and Head, Department of Medicine.

The language of this booklet is very simple and it is easy for the undergraduate students to follow. Echocardiograms are excellent. This book is clinically oriented and will be of a great help while understanding ECGs during the ward experience.

I congratulate Dr Pazare and Department of Medicine for providing this wonderful handbook to the students.

Best wishes

auSupe

Avinash Supe
Director (ME and MII)

Preface

It is difficult for the undergraduate students to read and understand electrocardiogram from various textbooks. They have too many subjects and vast topics to cover in short time. They also have to prepare for the postgraduate entrance examination in addition to their internship work. Hence, this short book is prepared keeping in mind the scarcity of time for undergraduates. This book summarizes important information on ECG and it is as per requirement of undergraduate curriculum. It is also a useful, handy booklet for general practitioners and postgraduates and faculty of other specialty and superspecialty (other than medicine and cardiology). This booklet serves handy information to all doctors as well as undergraduate students preparing for examination. It contains illustrative and simple ECGs which can be interpreted easily. This book revises knowledge in short time. I hope all the doctors will preserve this book for their life. I also hope this book will serve the purpose for which it is prepared.

Amar R Pazare

Contents

Foreword by Avinash Supe   v

Preface   vii

1. Introduction   1

2. Normal ECG   2

3. How to read ECG   3

4. Hypokalemia   5

5. Hyperkalemia   6

6. Arrhythmia   7

7. Sinus tachycardia   8

8. Sinus bradycardia   9

9. Paroxysmal supraventricular tachycardia   10

10. Atrial flutter   11

11. Atrial fibrillation   12

12. Idioventricular and accelerated idioventricular rhyth   14

13. Ventricular tachycardia   16

14. Ventricular fibrillation   18

15. Extrasystole   19

16. Atrioventricular block   21

17. Pre-excitation syndrome   24

18. Bundle branch block   26

19. Chamber hypertrophy   28

20. Ischemic heart disease   31

21. Pacemaker   33

    Index   35

Chapter 1

Introduction

Electrocardiogram (ECG) is the process of recording the electrical activity of the heart over a period of time using electrodes placed on the skin. These electrodes detect the tiny electrical changes on the skin that arise from the heart muscle's electrophysiologic pattern of depolarizing during each heartbeat. In a conventional 12-lead ECG, 4 electrodes are placed on the patient's limbs and 6 chest leads on the anterior surface of the chest. Thus ECG records 6 limb leads, i.e. lead I, II, III, aVR, aVL, and aVF which records electrical activity in lateral plane and 6 chest leads (V1–V6) record in vertical plane. ECG records on graph papers which move at the speed of 25 small boxes/second (1500 boxes/minute). Height of 1 small box is 1 mm and width is 0.04 second. Healthy heart has an orderly progression of depolarization that starts with pacemaker cells in the sinoatrial node, spreads out through the atrium, passes through the atrioventricular node down into the bundle of His and into the Purkinje fibers, spreading down throughout the ventricles. This orderly pattern of depolarization gives rise to the characteristic ECG tracing. ECG is used to measure the rate and rhythm of heart, the size and position of the heart chambers, the presence of any damage to the heart's muscle cells or conduction system, the effects of cardiac drugs, and the function of implanted pacemakers.

Normal ECG

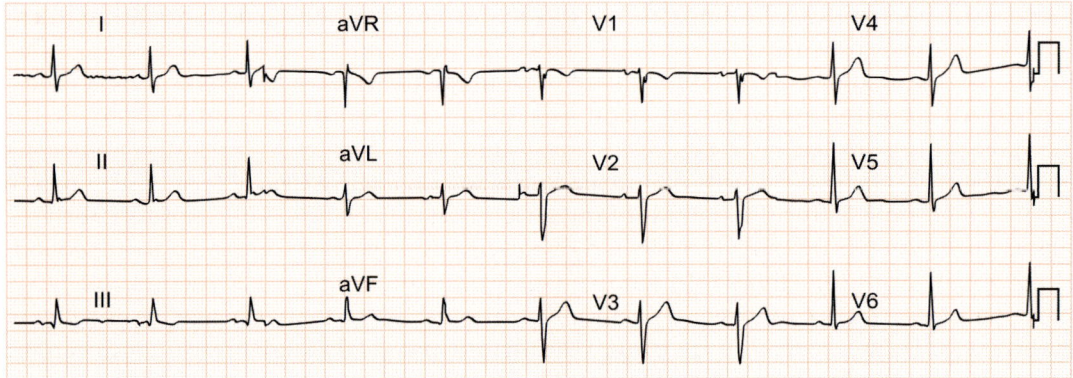

Graph showing normal ECG

How to Read ECG

1. **Heart rate:** It is calculated by formula (1500/no. of small boxes in RR interval). Heart rate in above ECG is calculated as 1500/25 = 60 beat/minute. Paper speed is 25 mm/second, hence 1 minute will have 1500 (60 × 25) small squares. This means 1500 small square denotes 1 minute.

2. **Regular:** All P, QRS complexes occurring at regular interval.

3. **Rhythm:** Normal ECG will have sinus rhythm, i.e. all QRS complexes are preceded by P wave of same configuration in same lead (above ECG). Positive P wave in all limb leads except aVR.

4. **Axis:** It is the direction of travelling of the electrical impulse. Normal Axis of P, QRS, and T wave is around 60 degrees. All limb leads record impulse in the direction of impulse except aVR which records in the opposite to the direction of impulse, hence normal ECG, all limb leads will have positive P, QRS complexes and T wave except aVR which shows negative complexes. Positive R waves in lead I and III suggest normal axis (as in above ECG). Positive R in lead I and negative R in lead III suggest left axis and negative R in lead I and positive R in lead III suggest right axis. In above ECG lead aVF shows nearly equal height of R and S wave (equiphasic complexes). It suggests axis is perpendicular to lead aVF and lead I is perpendicular to lead aVF. If axis is towards lead I, then lead I should have positive deflection (which is seen in above ECG and axis is zero degree) and if lead I would have shown negative deflection, then axis is exactly opposite of lead I (180 degrees). All limb leads are perpendicular to particular lead. Lead I is perpendicular to aVF, lead II is perpendicular to aVL and lead III is perpendicular to aVR. Normal axis is from 0 to + 90 degree, left axis is from 0 to –30 degrees (left ventricular hypertrophy) and right axis is from +90 to +120 degrees (right ventricular hypertrophy). Abnormal right axis is +120 to 180 degrees (left posterior hemiblock, LPHB), abnormal left axis is from –30 to –90 degrees (left anterior hemiblock, LAHB) and axis from – 90 to 180 degrees is indeterminate axis (axis of LAHB or LPHB may fall in that area).

5. **P wave:** Positive P wave prior to QRS complexes seen all the leads except aVR. Normal height of P wave is ≤ 2.5 mm and width ≤ 0.10 second.

6. **PR interval** (starting of P wave to starting of QRS complex)**:** PR interval varies from 0.12 second to 0.20 second. Usually this time is required for the impulse to travel from SA node to the myocardium via AV node, bundle of His, left and right bundle and Purkinje system. PR interval < 0.12 second suggests impulse has bypass normal conducting system (pre-excitation syndrome) and >0.20 second suggest heart blocks.

7. **QRS complex:** Normal duration of QRS complex is ≤ 0.10 second. Duration of > 0.10 second suggest bundle branch block, ventricular extrasystole or WPW syndrome.

8. **ST segment and T wave changes:** Normally ST segment is at the level of TP line. Upward or downward deviation of ST segment suggests myocardial ischemia. T wave is usually positive in all the leads except aVR. T wave inversion also suggests myocardial ischemia.

9. **Chamber hypertrophy:** Discussed elsewhere.

10. **Miscellaneuos:** Tall T wave (hyperkalemia), U wave (additional positive wave after T wave) (hypokalemia)

Hypokalemia

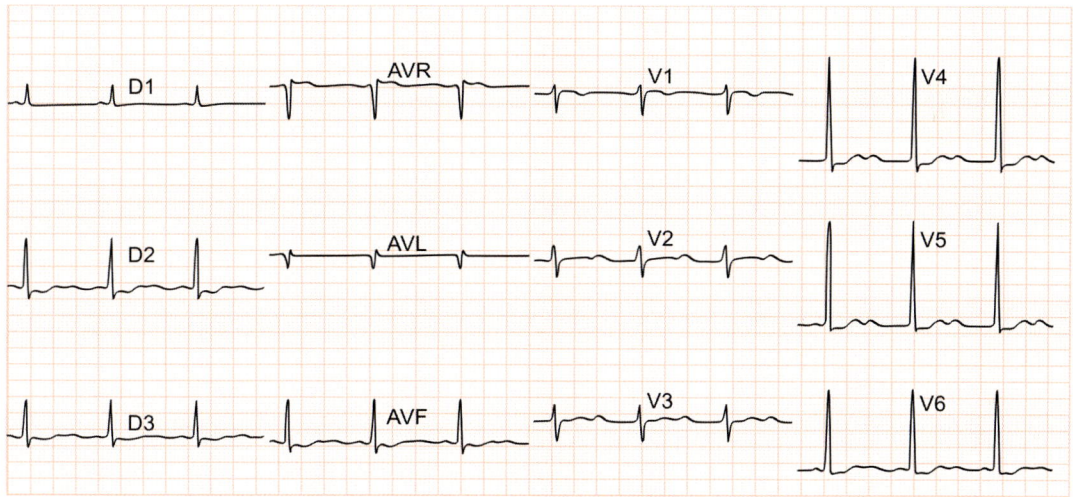

ECG shows U wave (hypokalemia)

Hyperkalemia

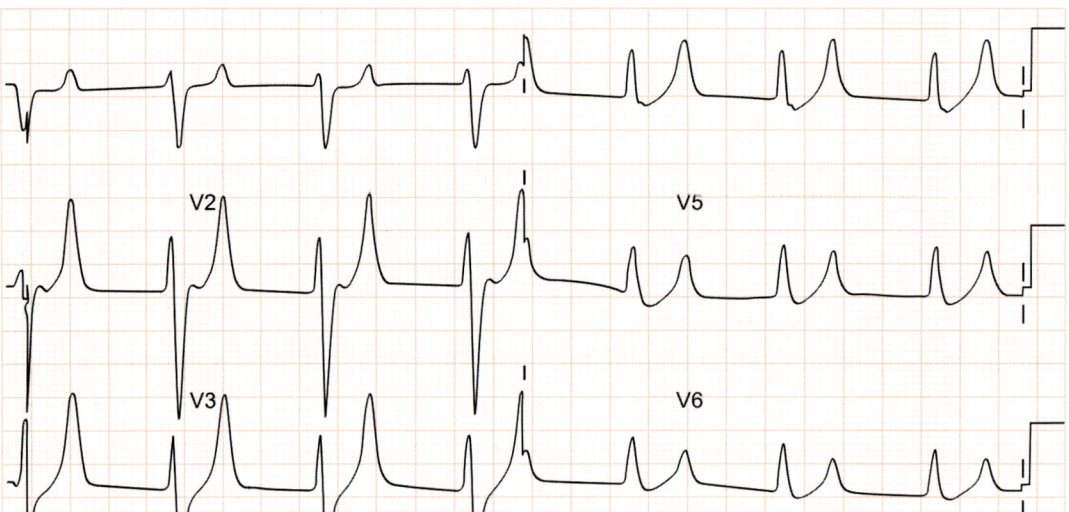

ECG shows tall tainted T wave (hyperkalemia)

Arrhythmia

Heart has a unique electrical apparatus called sino-atrial (SA) node which forms the impulse at regular interval throughout life of the person. And well-developed conducting system of the heart helps the impulse to travel to myocardium and maintain the muscle contraction within desirable limits. Thus SA node and conducting system maintain heart rate within the range of 60–100 beats/minute, thus maintain the cardiac output. In a few circumstances SA node may stop, increase or decrease its function, or conducting system misconducts or does not conduct the impulses to myocardium. It results in an arrhythmias or heart blocks. Sometimes other part of cardiac tissue may also act as a pacemaker.

SUPRAVENTRICULAR ARRHYTHMIAS

There may be stoppage or increase or decrease in SA node activity or there may be abnormal impulse formation in atrial tissue.

SINUS ARRHYTHMIA

It is usually a physiological phenomenon. It is more frequently seen in young people compared to older people. There is a variation in heart rate, i.e. there is increase in heart rate during inspiration compared to expiration. There is decrease in venous return (trapping of blood in the lung during inspiration due to more negative pressure) to left side of heart during inspiration and to maintain cardiac output heart rate increases. No treatment required for this condition.

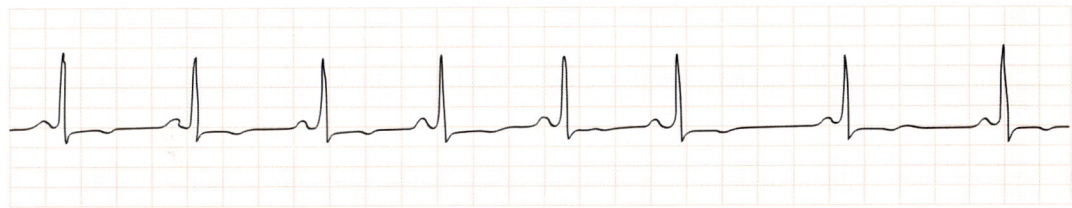

ECG shows variation in heart rate (range from 65 to 100 beat/minute) with normal P and QRS complexes

Chapter 7

Sinus Tachycardia

Sinus node fires more than 100 beat/minute and maximum rate can go up to 200 beats/minute during strenuous exercise. It may cause palpitation but person is usually hemodynamically stable. ECG usually shows a heart rate of 100–160 with preceding P wave.

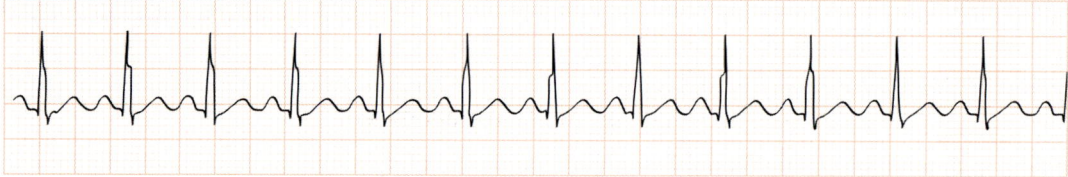

ECG shows sinus tachycardia at rate of 125 beats/minute

QRS complexes may be narrow or wide depending upon block at bundle branches. This tachycardia is usually occurs as compensation for a requirement of body demand. Demand is increased with exercise, fever, heart failure, thyrotoxicosis, etc. There is no need to treat this tachycardia. Treatment may require for treating the basic conditions like paracetamol for fever or digitalis for heart failure. Propranolol (beta-blockers) may require in symptomatic tachycardia with thyrotoxicosis or anxiety neurosis in addition to the treatment of basic conditions.

Chapter 8

Sinus Bradycardia

Heart rate is less than 60 beats/minute referred to as sinus bradycardia. It may be physiological (athletes or sleep), or pathological or may be due to side effect of drugs (beta-blockers, digitalis). Pathological conditions include hypothermia, hypothyroidism, increased intracranial pressure, intrinsic disease of the SA node (e.g. sick sinus syndrome) or it may be secondary to infections like diphtheria, acute rheumatic fever, viral myocarditis.

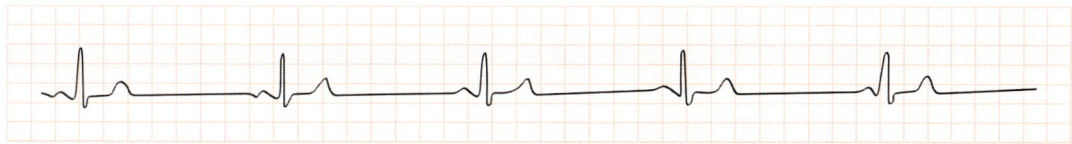

ECG shows sinus bradycardia at rate of 36 beats/minute

The decreased heart rate can cause a decreased cardiac output resulting in symptoms such as lightheadedness, dizziness, hypotension, vertigo, and syncope. Most cases treatment is not required but in symptomatic patient, atropine, isoprenaline or atrial pacemaker may be required. ECG shows heart rate < 60 beats/ minute and every beat is preceded by P wave with regular RR interval.

Chapter 9

Paroxysmal Supraventricular Tachycardia

Heart rate ranges between 120 and 240 beats/minute. This arrhythmia is transient and may revert back to normal without intervention. Usually there is no underlying heart disease. Paroxysmal supraventricular tachycardia (PSVT) is due to a reentered phenomenon. Critically placed atrial premature contraction (APC) can trigger reentered tachycardia through AV node. Only one path in AV node recovers after APC which allows impulse to pass through it and retrogradely enters other path. This results in perpetuating reentered tachycardia. Patient may present as syncope or pre-syncope, hypotension, palpitation, sweating and rarely pulmonary edema. ECG shows heart rate between 120 and 240 beats/minute with negative P wave in lead II, III and aVF (atria stimulates through retrograde impulse from AV node) and narrow QRS complexes.

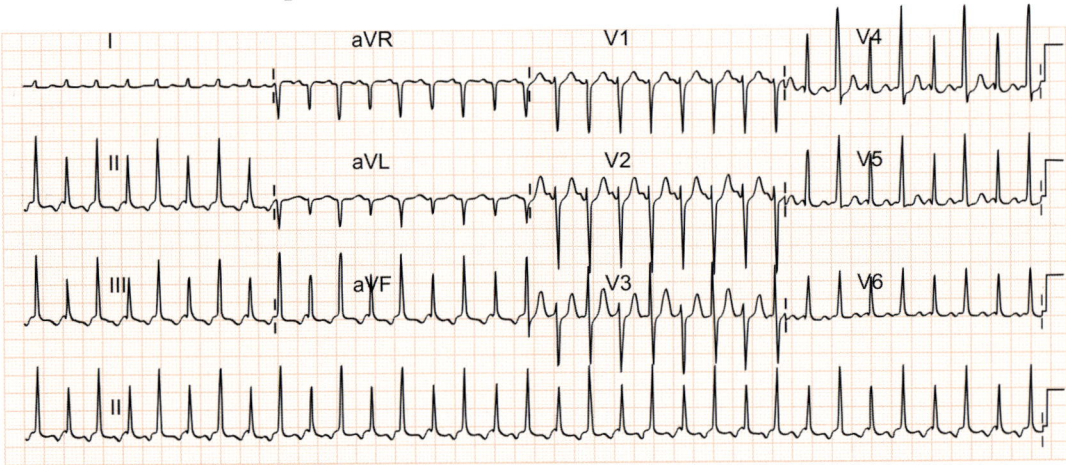

ECG shows PSVT at the rate of 215/minute with retrograde P wave in II, III, aVF and narrow QRS complex

Acute management of PSVT includes controlling the rate and preventing hemodynamic collapse. If the patient is hypotensive or unstable, immediate cardioversion is performed. If the patient is stable, then vagal maneuvers like eyeball pressure or carotid body massage may be tried or adenosine or calcium channel blockers or beta-blockers may be used.

Chapter 10

Atrial Flutter

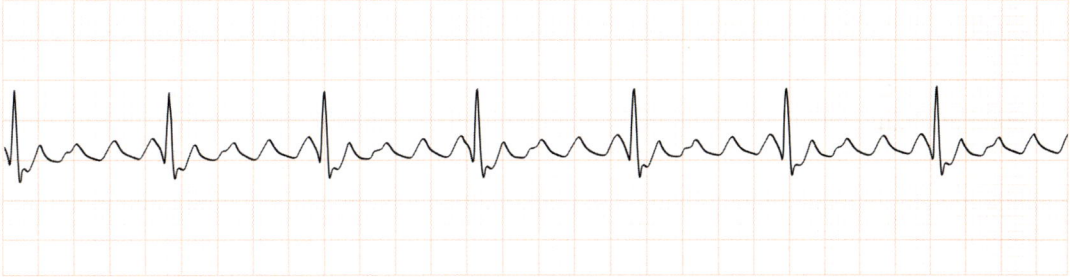

ECG shows atrial flutter (atrial rate of 300/minute and ventricular rate of 75/minute with 4:1 block)

Atrial flutter: Atrial rate is more than 200 beats/minute and show sawtooth appearance of P wave in ECG. There is a physiological block at AV node which blocks multiple atrial contractions. This gives rise to mobitz II type of heart block. Therefore, heart rate and pulse rate are maintained. These persons are usually asymptomatic with no hemodynamic instability. Usually this arrhythmia does not require any intervention except for clot in atria for which anticoagulation may be required.

Chapter 11

Atrial Fibrillation

Atrial rate is more than 350/minute with no definite visible P wave seen in surface ECG but fibrillatory waves may be visible. Mechanism of atrial fibrillation (AF) is usually ectopic (multifocal) or rarely it can be reentry. Atrial fibrillation (AF) may be coarse (mitral stenosis), fine (thyrotoxicosis) or sometime straight baseline (irregularly irregular placed QRS complexes are the only evidences of AF in such cases). Changing block is the reason for irregular and lower ventricular rate. Etiology of AF includes rheumatic heart disease, ischemic heart diseases, thyrotoxicosis, degenerative heart disease, cardiomyopathy, hypertension, syphilitic heart disease or lone (idiopathic).

Patient may present with palpitation (rapid ventricular rate), or systemic or pulmonary embolization (clot in LA or RA) or rarely asymptomatic. On examination pulse is irregularly irregular with apex pulse deficit of more than 12/minute and absent 'a' wave in JVP. If patient has additional diagnosis of mitral stenosis (MS), then some auscultatory finding of MS will be modified (changing intensity of M1, disappearance of presystolic accentuation of mid-diastolic murmur). Regular pulse in a diagnose case of AF is not a good sign. It probably suggests complete heart block (digoxin toxicity).

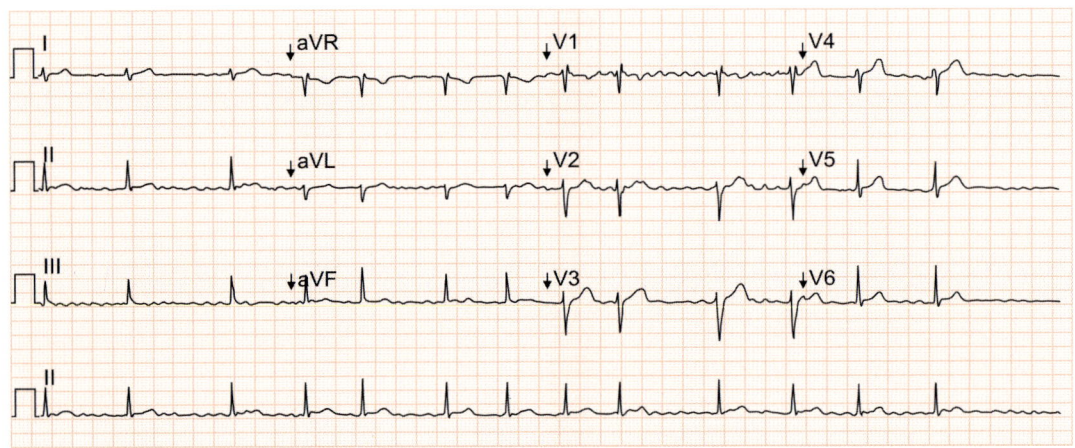

ECG shows fibrillatory waves, narrow QRS complexes and changing RR interval (AF)

Usually treatment is not required when ventricular rate is maintained below 100/minute. Drugs like digoxin, diltezam, amadarone may be used to control heart rate. Long-standing diseases like mitral valve disease, cardiomyopathy usually have large left atria. Hence rhythm control in these patients is not rewarding. However, AF of shorter duration, rhythm control may be warranted. And quinidine, or electrical conversion may be used for rhythm control. Withhold digoxin and heparinise the patient at least a week prior to electrical conversion if patient has a clot in LA.

Chapter 12

Idioventricular and Accelerated Idioventricular Rhythm

Ventricular rate up to 50 beats/minute is called **idioventricular rhythm** (IVR) and ventricular rate of 50–110 is called **accelerated idioventricular rhythm (AIVR)**. There are wide QRS complexes (>0.12 sec, often >0.16) seconds with no prior P waves. This is a benign arrhythmia and can occur in normal healthy individuals. AIVR is often a clue to certain underlying conditions, like myocardial ischemia-reperfusion—digoxin toxicity, and cardiomyopathies. There may be sinus fire, rate

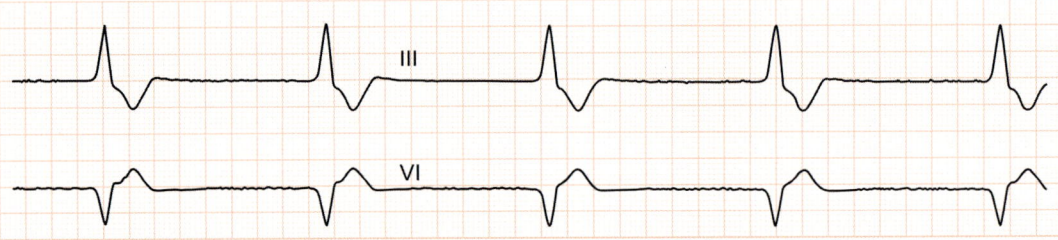

ECG shows ventricular rate of 35/minute (IVR)

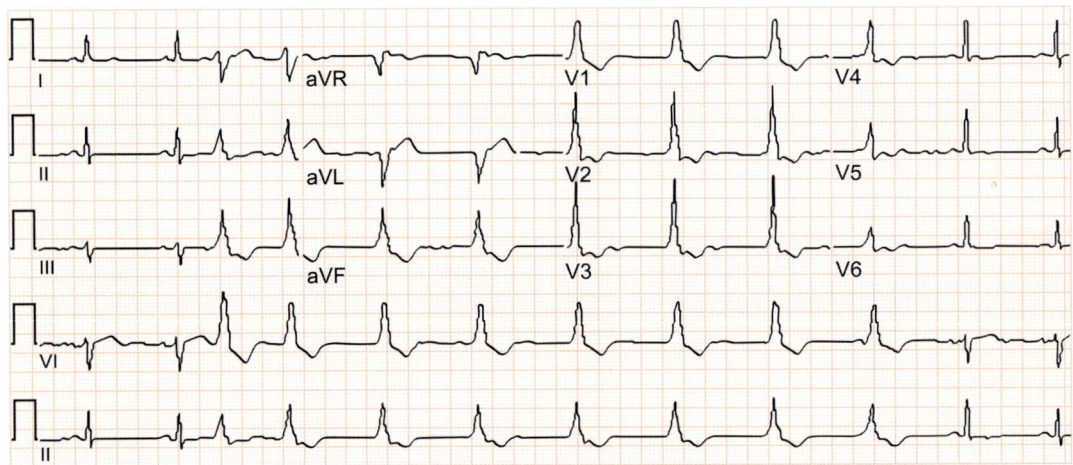

ECG shows AIVR at rate of 75/minute

of which is less than ventricular rhythm. Sinus P may be visible on surface electrocardiogram. There may be retrograde conduction of impulses to atria. Usually no treatment is required for this condition. If there is severe bradycardia and causing symptoms (hypotension, syncope, giddiness), then treatment in the form of pacemaker may be required.

Chapter 13

Ventricular Tachycardia

Ventricular tachycardia (VT) is defined as a sequence of three or more ventricular beats and usually ventricular rate is 110–250/minute. It often originates from area around old scar tissue in the heart, e.g. after myocardial infarction or it occurs in conditions like electrolyte disturbances and ischemia or may be idiopathic. The cardiac output is often compromised during VT resulting in hypotension and loss of consciousness. VT is a medical emergency as it can terminate into ventricular fibrillation and cardiac arrest. Although VT is often associated with cardiac disease but short non-sustained VT can occur during exercise or healthy individuals, which has good prognosis. It is categorized as follows:

- **Non-sustained VT:** Three or more ventricular beats with a maximal duration of 30 seconds.
- **Sustained VT:** VT of more than 30 seconds duration (or less if treated by electrocardioversion within 30 seconds).
- **Monomorphic VT:** All ventricular beats have the same configuration.
- **Polymorphic VT:** The ventricular beats have a changing configuration. It usually occurs due to prolong QT interval (torsade de pointes)

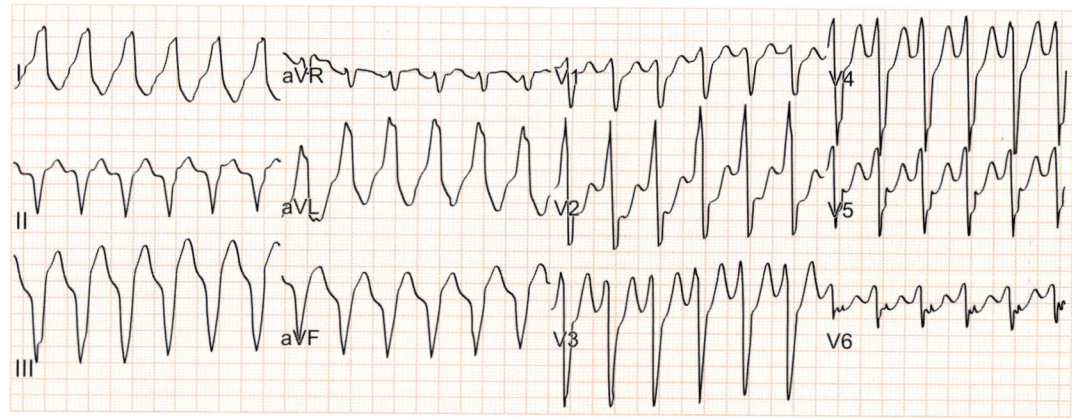

ECG shows monomorphic VT at rate of 150/minute

- **Biphasic VT:** A ventricular tachycardia with a QRS complex that alternates from beat to beat. It is associated with digoxin intoxication and long QT syndrome.

Ventricular tachycardia can be differentiated from supraventricular tachycardia (SVT) with wide QRS complexes (LBBB, RBBB, WPW syndrome). Prior P wave before QRS complexes present before SVT but sometimes it is difficult to differentiate between two types of arrhythmia.

TORSADE DE POINTES

Torsade de pointes is an uncommon and distinctive form of polymorphic ventricular tachycardia (VT) characterized by a gradual change in the amplitude and twisting of the QRS complexes (twisting of the points) around the isoelectric line. It is associated with a prolonged QT interval, which may be congenital or acquired. Congenital causes include Jervell and Lange-Nielsen syndrome (i.e. congenitally long QT associated with congenital deafness) and the Romano Ward syndrome (i.e. isolated prolongation of QT interval). Both of these syndromes are associated with sudden death due to ventricular fibrillation. Acquired conditions include hypokalemia, hypomagnesemia, antiarrhythmic drugs (quinidine, procainamide, disopyramide, encainide, flecainide, sotalol, amiodarone), antihistamines (astemizole and terfenadine) alone or in combination with azole antifungal drugs or the macrolides. Torsade usually occurs in bursts that are not sustained; thus, the rhythm strip usually shows the patient's baseline QT prolongation.

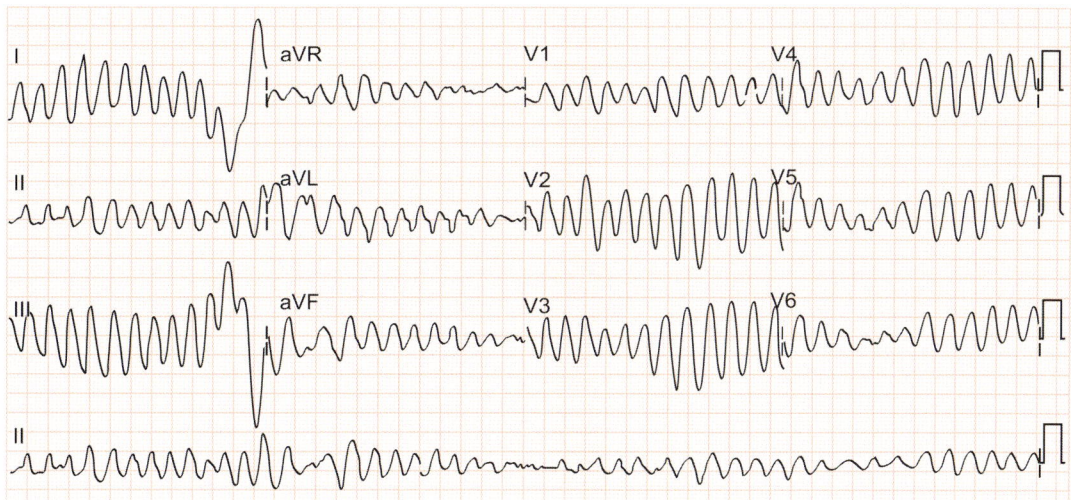

ECG shows torsade de pointes

Chapter 14

Ventricular Fibrillation

Ventricular fibrillation (VF) is a cause of cardiac arrest and sudden cardiac death. The ventricular muscle fibres contract randomly causing a complete failure of ventricular function.

VF is most often associated with coronary artery disease and as a terminal event. VF may be due to acute myocardial infarction (MI) or ischaemia, or occur because of a chronic infarction scar. Rarely it may occur in the pre-excitation syndrome or electrical shock caused by accidental contact with improperly grounded equipment. There may be history suggestive of coronary artery disease, cardiomyopathy, valvular heart disease, myocarditis, congenital heart disease, long QT syndrome, Wolff-Parkinson-White (WPW) syndrome or Brugada's syndrome. Management includes defibrillation (electrical cardioversion).

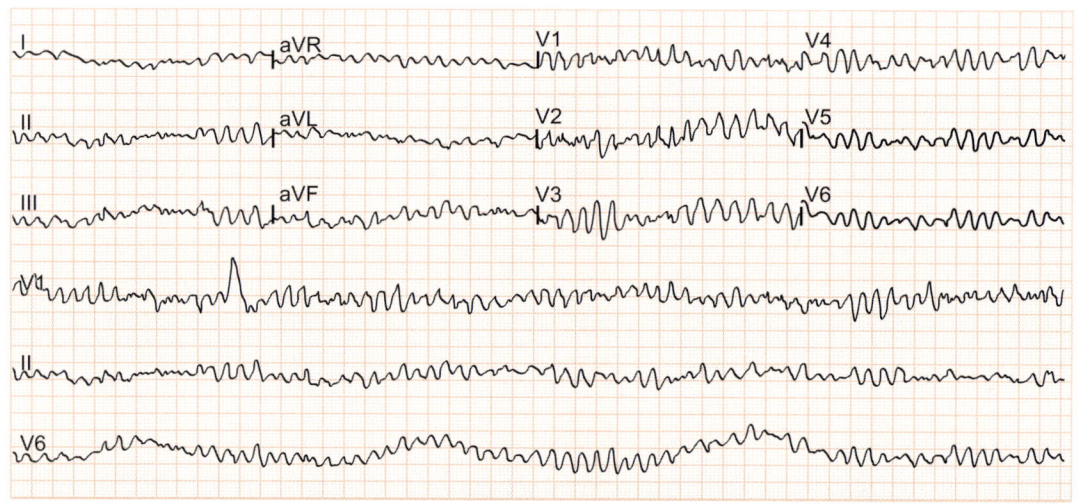

ECG shows ventricular fibrillation

Chapter 15

Extrasystole

Extrasystole is a premature cardiac contraction that is independent of the normal rhythm and arises outside the sinoatrial node. Since the heart muscle remains unexcitable for some time after every contraction, the next normal impulse usually blocked. Hence there is pause before next contraction (compensatory pause). Complete compensatory pause present in ventricular extrasystole while incomplete in supraventricular extrasystole. Atrial extrasystole shows different P' compared to sinus beat with marrow QRS complexes. Ventricular extrasystoles have wide and bizarre QRS complexes with no prior P waves. Nodal extrasystoles have narrow QRS complexes with absent or negative P' in lead II, III, aVF. Extrasystoles may be single or multiple, and they may occur chaotically or with a certain rhythm. For example, after every normal contraction there is an extrasystole called bigeminy or after 2 normal contraction there is an extrasystole called trigeminy. Sometimes several extrasystoles occur in succession. Interpolated extrasystole is a contraction taking place between two normal heartbeats.

Extrasystole can occur in a healthy person of any age, but are more prevalent in the elderly and in men without any known cause. But certain other conditions like IHD, Cardiomyopathy, Alcohol, drugs (digoxin, or tricyclic antidepressants, caffeine, cocaine), COPD, hypokalamia, smoking, stress, mitral valve prolapse, myocarditis may be responsible for extrasystole. An extrasystole is generally felt as a temporary sinking sensation, or an "interruption in the heart".

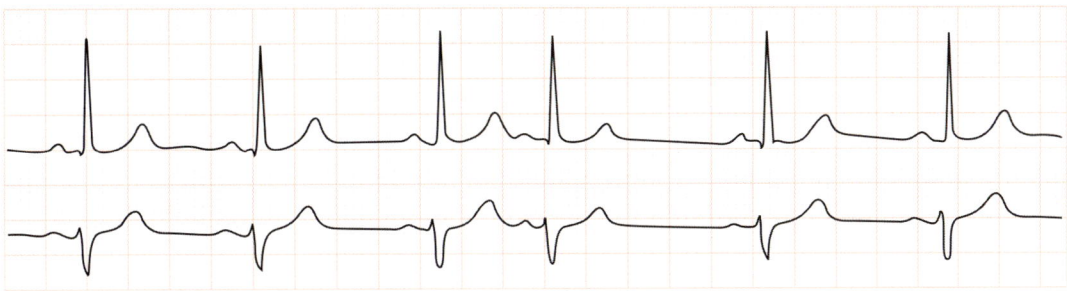

ECG shows 4th beat as atrial extrasystole (prior P' wave, narrow QRS complex and incomplete compensatory pause)

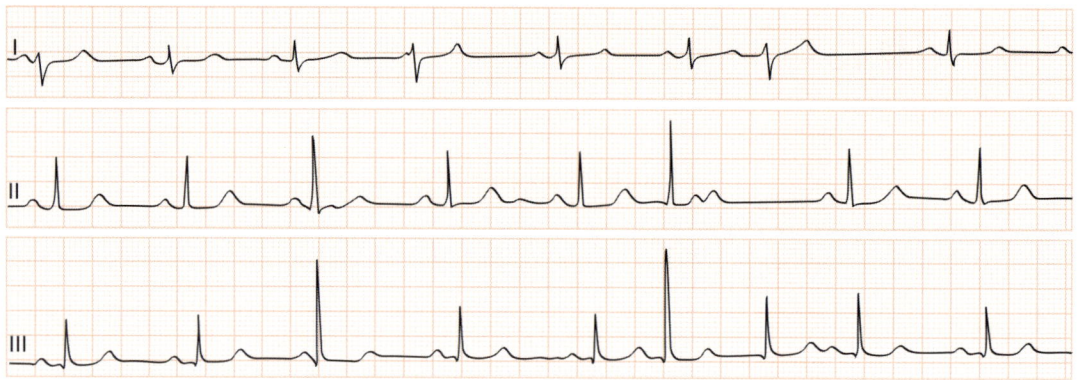

ECG shows 6th beat as nodal extrasystole (no P wave, narrow QRS complex and incomplete compensatory pause)

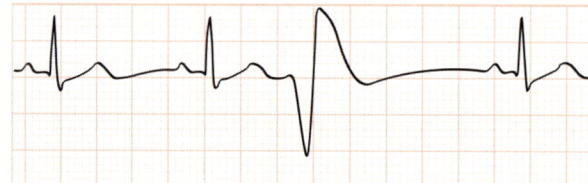

ECG shows ventricular extrasystole (no prior P wave, wide QRS complex and complete compensatory pause)

Ventricular extrasystole may be completely asymptomatic and discovered incidentally on a routine ECG or these are experienced as 'missed beats'. In structurally normal hearts, these are not dangerous. In the presence of significant structural heart disease, frequent ectopy marks an increased risk of sudden cardiac death, hence treatment is required. Rarely do these have the potential to induce ventricular fibrillation particularly if they coincide with the T wave of preceding beat (R on T phenomenon).

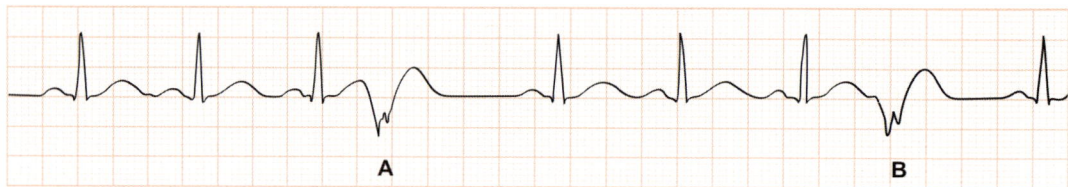

ECG shows R on T phenomenon

Chapter 16

Atrioventricular Block

Atrioventricular (AV) block is due to partial or complete interruption of impulse transmission from the atria to the ventricles. Common causes are ischemic heart disease (most likely right coronary disease), digoxin toxicity, beta blockers, viral myocarditis, rheumatic fever, infections mononucleosis, sarcoidosis, amyloidosis, degenerative heart disease (Lev's and Lenègre disease). It is classified as 1st, 2nd (Wenckebach's and Mobitz II) and 3rd degree AV block.

- **1st degree AV block:** PR interval is more than 0.20 seconds. Patient is asymptomatic and no treatment is required.

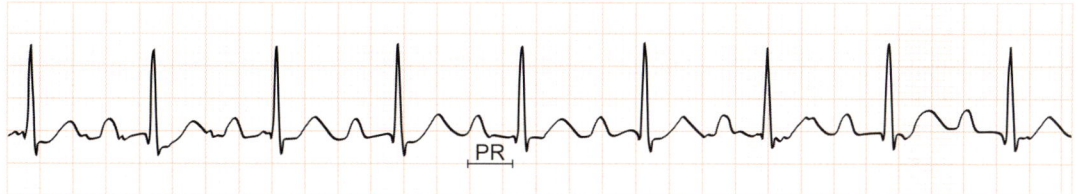

ECG shows PR interval of 0.28 seconds (1st degree AV block)

- **2nd degree (Wenckebach's phenomenon):** There is a gradual prolongation of PR interval followed by drop of one QRS complex. Hence AV block may be described as 3:2 (2 QRS complexes for 3 P waves) or 4:3 (3 QRS complexes for 4 P waves) or 5:4 (4 QRS complexes for 5 P waves) and so on. Patient is asymptomatic and no treatment is required.

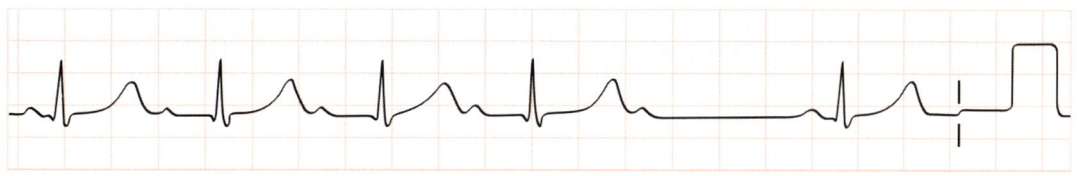

ECG shows gradual prolongation of PR interval with 5:4 type of block (Wenckebach's phenomenon)

- **2nd degree Mobitz II:** There is more severe block (multiple QRS complexes are blocked). There are multiple P waves for one QRS complex.

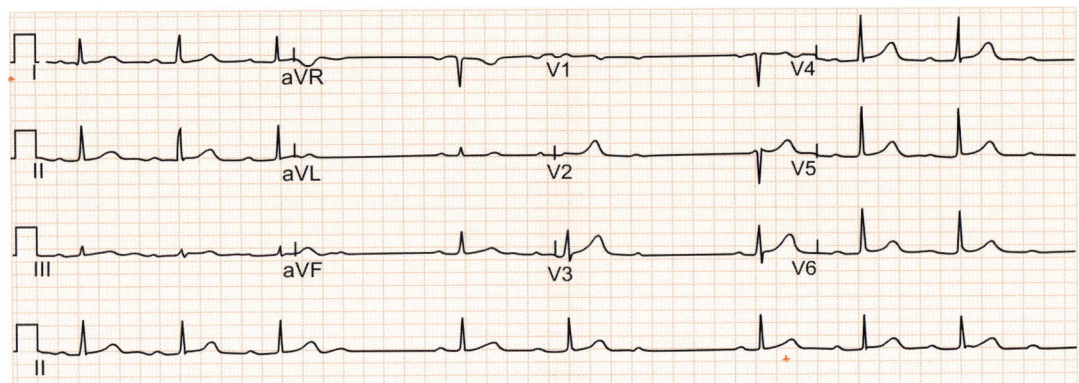

ECG shows 2:1 type of AV block (Mobitz II)

Hence AV block may be described as 2:1 (1 QRS complex for 2 P waves) or 3:1 (1 QRS complex for 3 P waves) or 4:1(1 QRS complex for 4 P waves) and so on. Patient may be symptomatic and symptoms depend on ventricular rate. Significant drop in ventricular rate may present as syncope and may require pacemaker.

- **3rd degree/complete heart block (CHB):** This is the severe form of AV nodal disease where the impulse from the atria does not transmit to the ventricle. Atria contract at its own rate (around 72 beat/min and regular) and ventricular

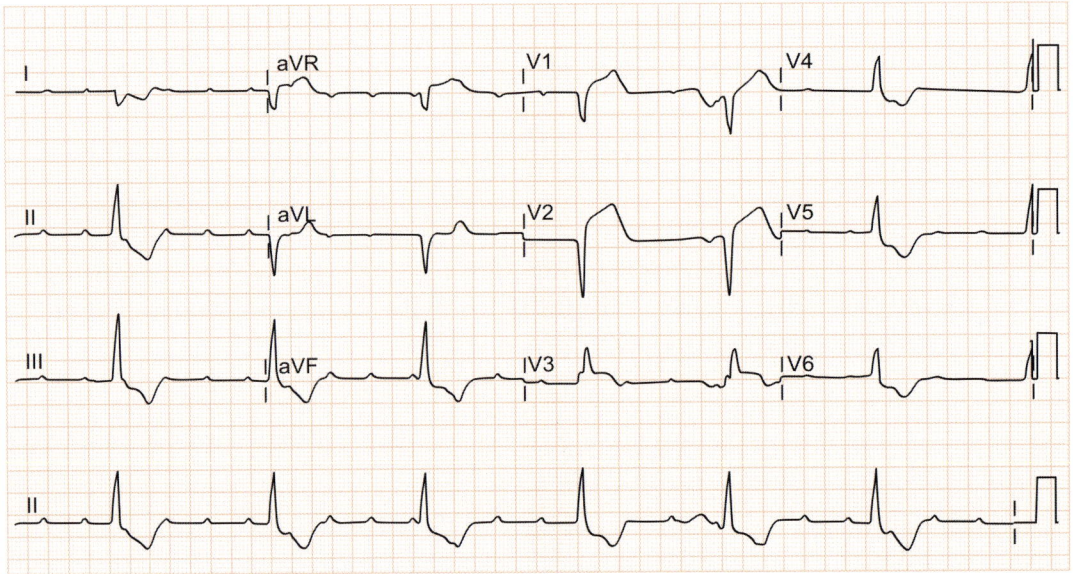

ECG shows atrial rate of 150 beats/minute regular and ventricular rate of 40 beats/minute regular and wide QRS complexes (CHB)

contracts at its own rate (30–40 beats/min and regular) and there is no relation of P to QRS complex on ECG. CHB may be congenital where ventricular rate is on higher side (around 60 beats/minute) with narrow QRS complexes. Focus of impulse is around fascicle and patient is asymptomatic. Acquired CHB has ventricular rate on lower side (around 40 beats/minute) with wide and bizarre QRS complexes. Focus of impulse in the ventricle. These patients are usually symptomatic in the form of syncope, Stokes-Adams syndrome. Permanent pacemaker is required for degenerative heart disease like Lev's and Lenègre disease while temporary pacemaker may require for other conditions.

Chapter 17

Pre-excitation Syndrome

Wolff Parkinson-White (WPW) syndrome: WPW syndrome is caused by the presence of an abnormal accessory electrical conduction pathway between the atria and the ventricles. Electrical signals traveling down this abnormal pathway (known as the bundle of Kent) may stimulate the ventricles to contract prematurely, resulting in a unique type of supraventricular tachycardia referred to as an atrioventricular re entrant tachycardia. It is manifested as short PR interval (impulse passing through Kent fibre bypassing normal conducting system), a delta wave (slurred upstroke in the QRS complex, ventricular muscles stimulated through Kent fibre with muscle to muscle conduction), broad QRS complex but normal QT interval and T wave inversion.

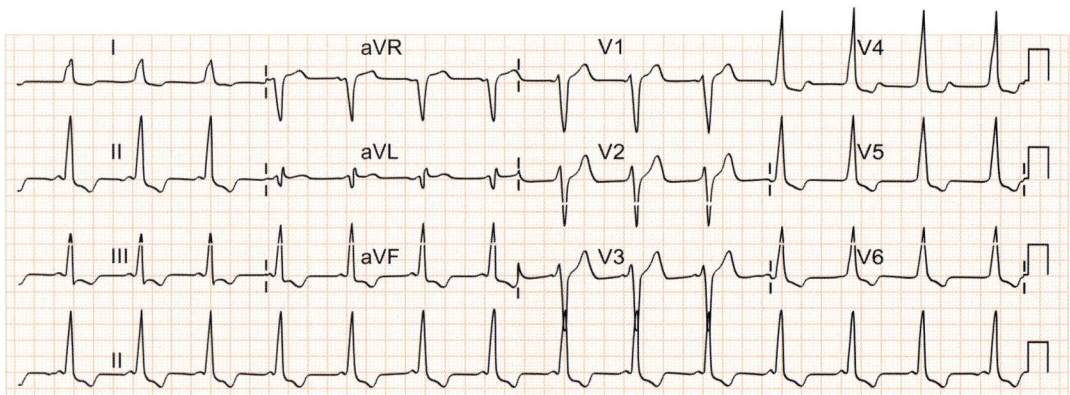

ECG shows short PR interval (0.10 seconds), delta wave on upstroke of R wave, broad QRS complexes and T wave inversion (WPW syndrome)

Lown-Ganong-Levine (LGL) syndrome: There is an accessory path connecting atria to bundle of His or left or right bundle (fiber of James). Hence it has only short PR interval with normal QRS complexes (without delta wave) and paroxysms of clinically-significant tachycardia. Individuals with a short PR interval found incidentally on ECG were once thought to have LGL syndrome. However, subsequent studies have shown that a short PR interval in the absence of symptomatic tachycardia is simply a benign ECG variant.

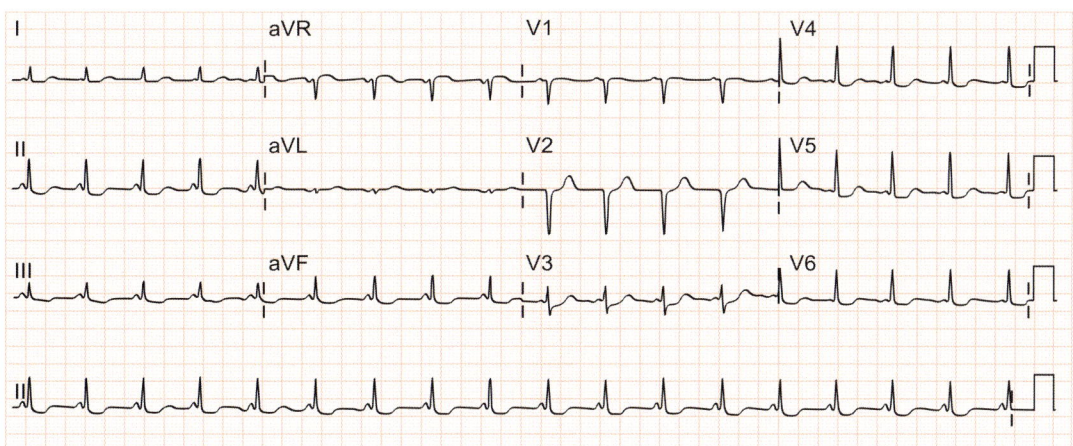

ECG shows short PR interval (0.08 second) with normal QRS complex at rate of 100 beats/minute

Chapter 18

Bundle Branch Block

In normal heart, supraventricular impulses conducted to right and left the ventricles through right and left bundles respectively. But in a few conditions one bundle is blocked and both the ventricles are activated by remaining bundles, thus ECG shows the abnormalities. And depending upon bundle blocked, it is referred to as right bundle branch block (RBBB) or left bundle branch block (LBBB). Etiology includes IHD, cardiomyopathy, myocarditis, hypertension, atrial septal defect and pulmonary embolism (especially RBBB), degenerative heart disease (Lev's and Lenègre's disease).

LBBB: As left bundle is blocked, left ventricle stimulated through right ventricle via right bundle by muscle to muscle conduction. Hence there will be wide QRS complex with rsR' pattern (M pattern) on left-sided lead (V5, V6). There will be deep and wide QRS complex in lead V1. Proper P wave is visible before each QRS complex. There is delayed left ventricle stimulation and without right ventricular apposing electrical activity which results in leftward axis.

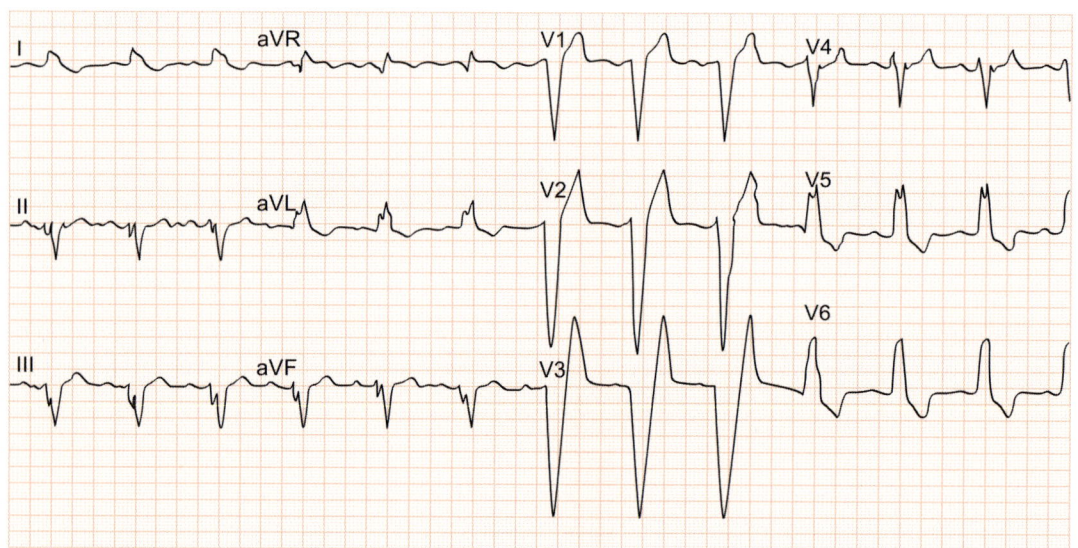

ECG shows left axis, wide and deep S wave in V1, rsR´ pattern (M pattern in V5, V6) (LBBB)

RBBB: As the right bundle is blocked, right ventricle stimulates through left ventricle via left bundle by muscle to muscle conduction. Hence there will be wide QRS complex with rsR′ pattern on right-sided lead (V1, V2). There will be wide S wave seen in lead V5, V6. Proper P wave is visible before every QRS complex. There will be no axis change as right ventricle is a weaker chamber compared to left.

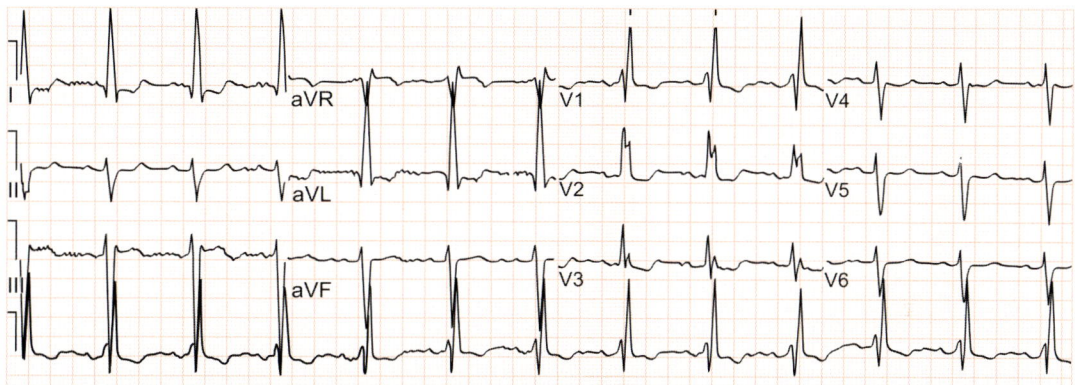

ECG shows rsR′ pattern in lead V1, wide S wave in V6 (RBBB)

Chapter 19

Chamber Hypertrophy

Any chamber may be enlarged or hypertrophied depending upon the excess of load it bears.

P mitrale (left atrial enlargement): Broad (more than 0.10 second) and notched P waves seen in many leads of the electrocardiogram and there may be a prominent late negative component to the P wave in lead V1, presumed to be characteristic of mitral valvular disease although other conditions like hypertension, cardiomyopathy may result in P mitrale.

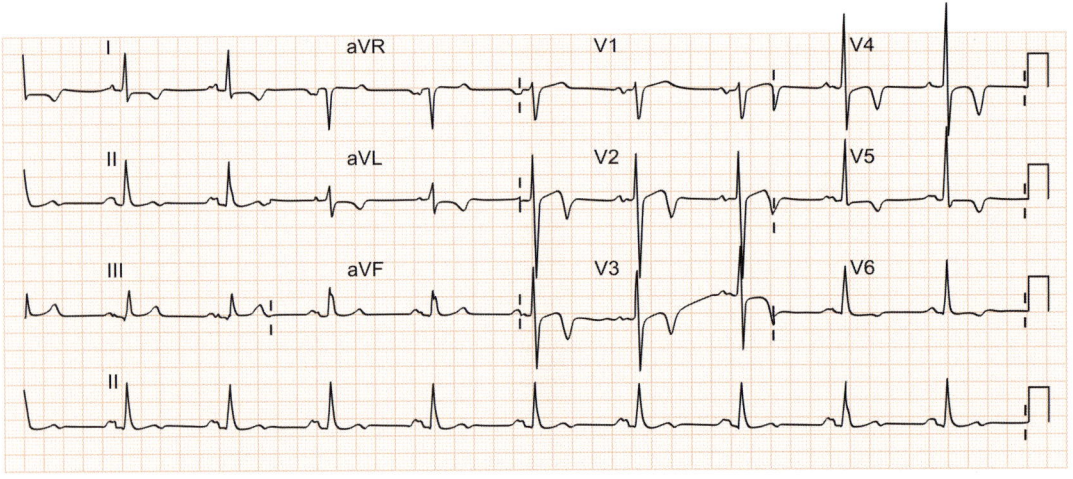

ECG shows broad (0.12 second) and bifid P waves more marked in lead II (P mitrale)

P Pulmonale (right atrial enlargement): There is tall and peaked P waves (height more than 2.5 mm, prominent in leads II, III, and aVF) and a prominent initial positive P wave component in V1, presumed to be characteristic of cor pulmonale (COPD or any chronic lung disease) although it may be seen in tricuspid stenosis. It may be seen transiently in acute exacerbations of bronchial asthmatic or pulmonary embolism.

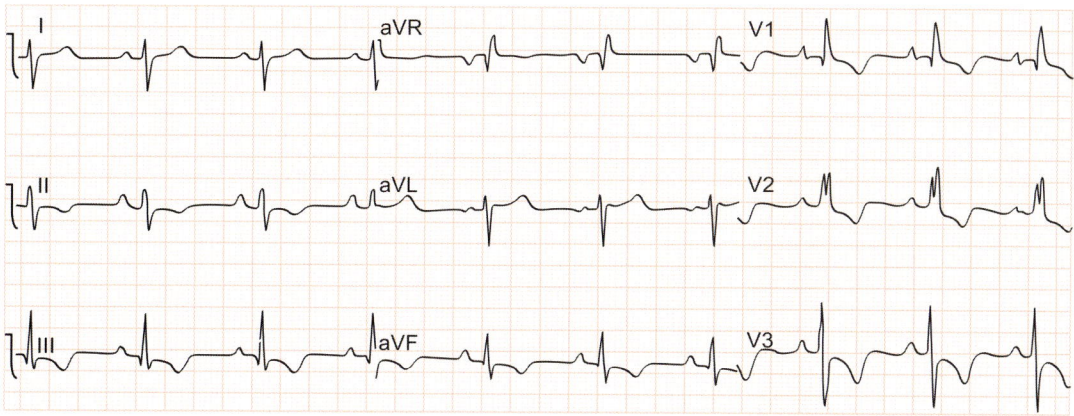

ECG shows tall peaked P wave (3 mm) prominent in lead II, III, aVF (P pulmonale)

LEFT VENTRICULAR HYPERTROPHY

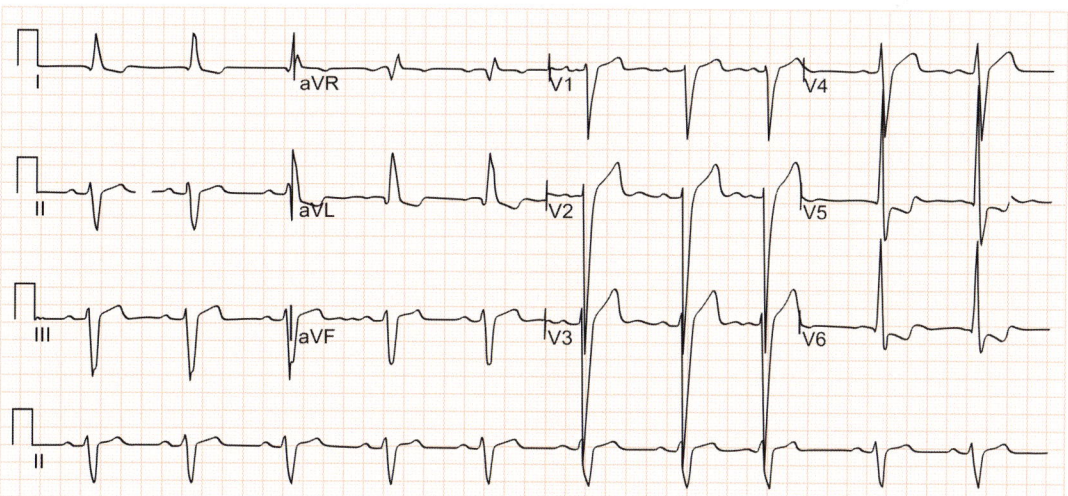

ECG shows left axis, SV2 + RV6 = 60 mm and ST depression and T wave inversion in V5, V6 (LVH)

Left ventricular hypertrophy (LVH): LVH can occur due to volume overload (mitral regurgitation, aortic regurgitation, thyrotoxicosis, anemia and beriberi) or pressure overload (hypertension, aortic stenosis, asymmetric septal hypertrophy). In ECG LVH diagnosed by voltage criteria (S wave in V1 + R in V5 or V6 or S wave in V2 + R in V6 ≥35 mm or R in V5, or V6 ≥25 mm) and left axis deviation. Additional finding like ST segment depression with T wave inversion in lateral leads I, aVL, V5, V6 may present in pressure overload conditions.

Right ventricular hypertrophy (RVH): RVH can present in conditions like pulmonary hypertension, tetralogy of Fallot, pulmonary stenosis, chronic obstructive pulmonary disease (COPD). ECG findings include right axis deviation, tall R-waves in V1(R:S >1) and deep S-waves in V5, V6.

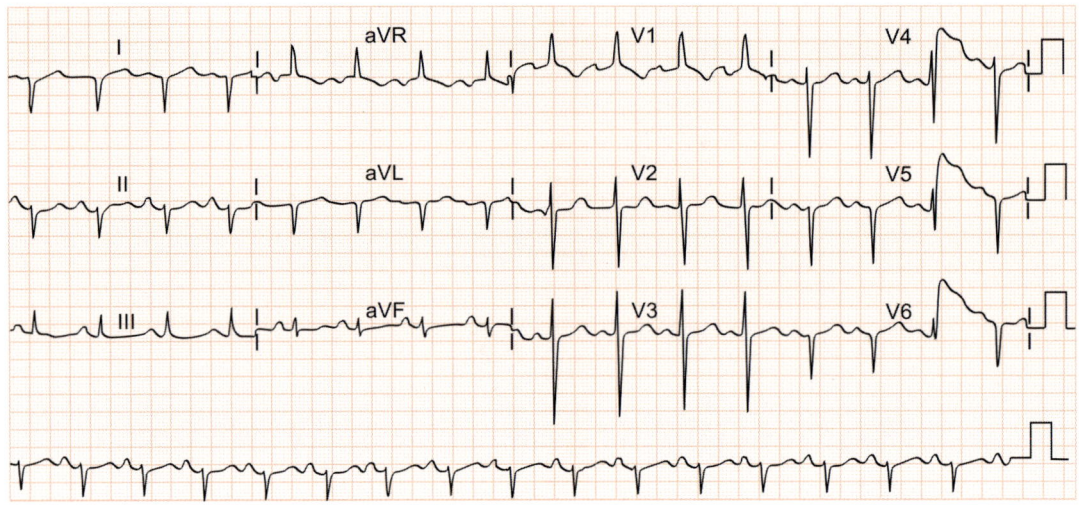

ECG shows right axis deviation, R wave in V1 and deep S wave in V5, V6 (RVH)

Chapter 20

Ischemic Heart Disease

Ischemia, most of the time is due to coronary artery disease, however, embolization to coronary artery may be rare cause of ischemia. Hypertension or aortic stenosis will result in left ventricular hypertrophy which demands more blood supply and it is not met with normal coronary artery which results in ischemia of myocardium. Depending upon severity of ischemia, ischemic heart disease (IHD) is classified as ischemia or infarction. Ischemia may be transient (angina pectoris, changes in ECG during chest pain), or prolong (ischemia, persistent ECG changes). ST, T wave changes in LVH are called strain pattern. There may be ST elevation myocardial infarction (STEMI) or non-STEMI (NSTEMI, symmetrical T wave inversion). Infarction can be Q wave infarction or non-Q wave infarction. Site of infarction can be judged on the basis of changes in specific leads. Changes in II, III, aVF suggest inferior wall involvement, V1– V4 suggests anterior wall involvement and changes in I, aVL, V5, V6 suggest lateral wall involvement. Sudden appearance of R wave in V1 (reciprocal changes) suggests posterior wall involvement.

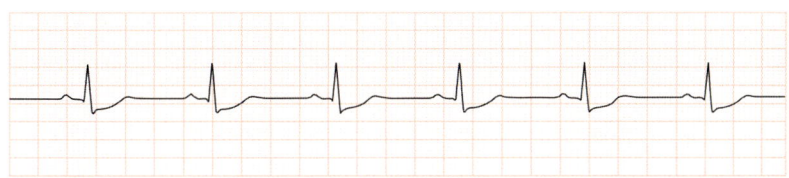

ECG shows ST segment depression (angina pectoris, or ischemia of myocardium)

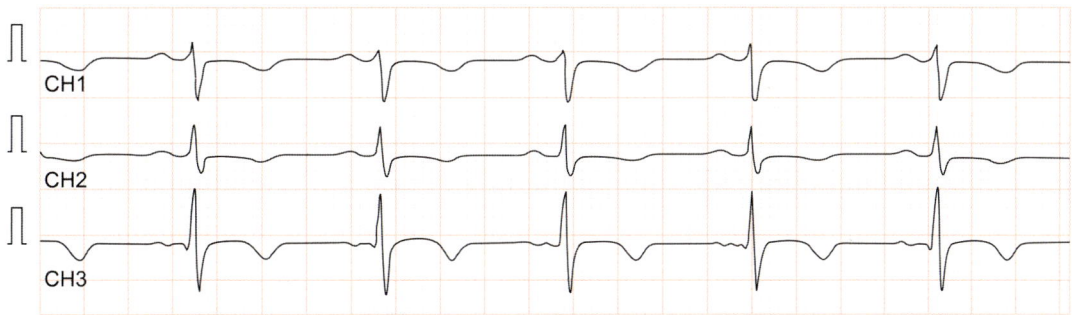

ECG shows symmetrical T wave inversion (NSTEMI)

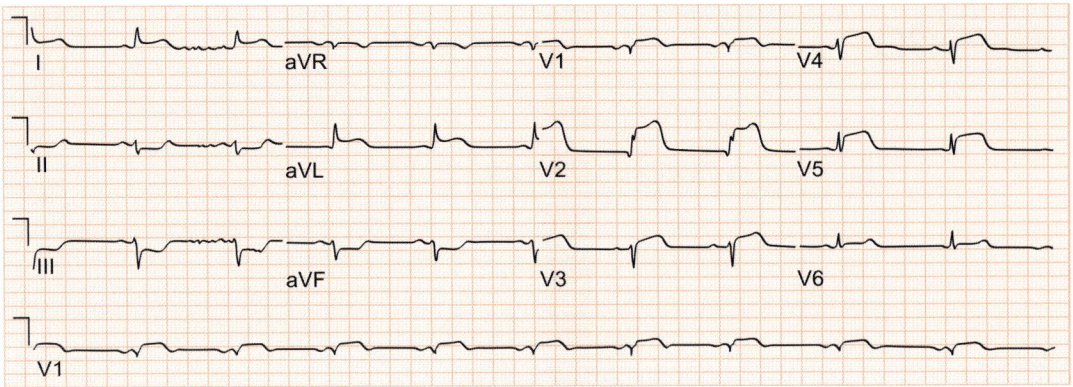

ECG shows ST segment elevation inV1–V5 (STEMI), ST segment depression in II, III, aVF (reciprocal changes)

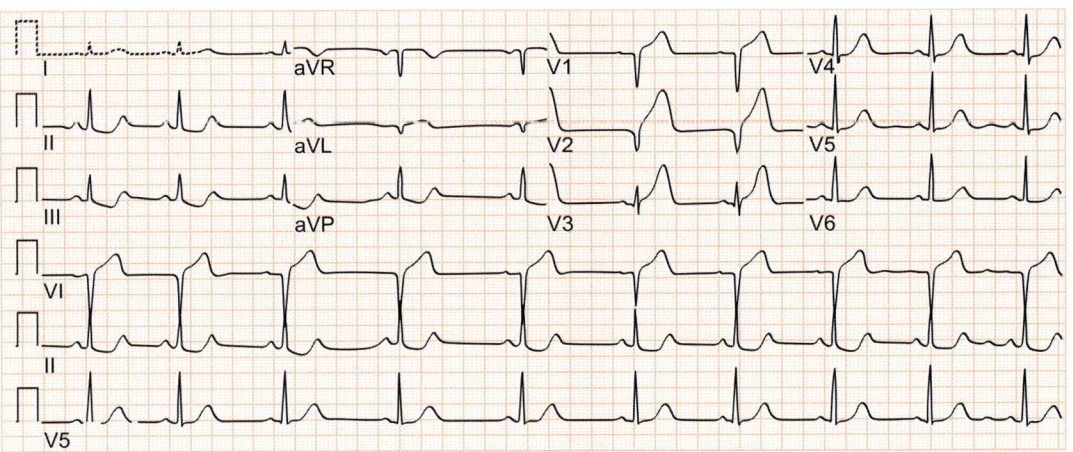

ECG shows Q wave in V1–V3 (Q wave infarction)

Chapter 21

Pacemaker

Cardiac pacemaker is a medical device implanted subcutaneously over chest in a subclavicular area and connected to right ventricular mass or rarely right atria (overdrive pacemaker) by electrical wires. It gives desired electrical impulses to heart so as heart contracts at normal rate and rhythm. The primary purpose of a pacemaker is to maintain an adequate heart rate, either because the heart's natural pacemaker is not fast enough, or because there is a block in the heart's electrical conduction system. Modern pacemakers are externally programmable and allow a cardiologist to select the optimum pacing modes for individual patients. Combined pacemaker and defibrillator in a single implantable device is also available. Newer pacemakers have multiple electrodes stimulating differing positions within the heart to improve synchronization of the lower chambers (ventricles) of the heart.

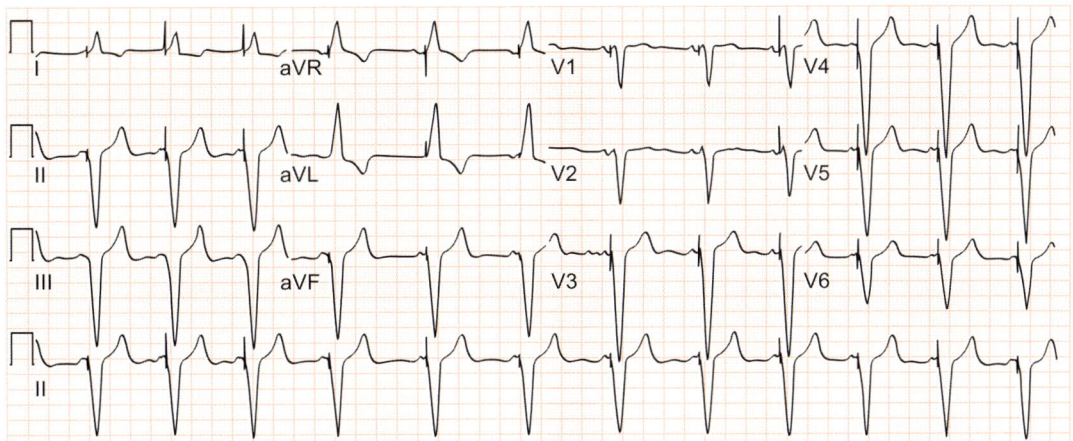

ECG shows vertical straight line before each QRS complex (pacemaker wire)

Index

12-Lead ECG 1
Accelerated idioventricular rhythm (AIVR) 14
Adenosine 10
Amadarone 13
Arrhythmias 7
Atrial fibrillation (AF) 12
Atrial flutter 11
Atrial premature contraction (APC) 10
Atrioventricular (AV) block 21
Axis 3

Bigeminy 19
Biphasic VT 17

Cardiac pacemaker 33
Chamber hypertrophy 4

Depolarization 1
Digoxin 13
Diltezam 13

ECG tracing 1
Extrasystole 19

Heart rate 3
Hyperkalemia 6
Hypokalemia 5

Idioventricular rhythm (IVR) 14
Ischemic heart disease (IHD) 31

Jervell syndrome 17

Lange-Nielsen syndrome 17
Left bundle branch block 26
Left ventricular hypertrophy 29

Lev's and Lenègre disease 21
Lown-Ganong-Levine (LGL) syndrome 24

Mitral stenosis 12
Mitral valve disease 13
Monomorphic VT 16

Nodal extrasystole 20
Non-sustained VT 16
Normal ECG 2

P mitrale 28
P pulmonale 28
P wave 3
Paroxysmal supraventricular tachycardia (PSVT) 10
Polymorphic VT 16
PR interval 4
Purkinje fibers 1

QRS complexes 4, 8

R on T phenomenon 20
Rhythm 3
Right bundle branch block 26
Right ventricular hypertrophy (RVH) 29
Romano Ward syndrome 17

Sino-atrial (SA) node 7
Sinus arrhythmia 7
Sinus bradycardia 9
Sinus fire 14
Sinus tachycardia 8
ST segment 4
Strenuous exercise 8

Supraventricular arrhythmias 7
Sustained VT 16

T wave changes 4
Thyrotoxicosis 12
Torsade de pointes 17
Trigeminy 19

Ventricular extrasystole 20
Ventricular tachycardia (VT) 16
Viral myocarditis 9

Wenckebach's and Mobitz II 21
Wolff-Parkinson-White (WPW) syndrome
    18, 24

Reader's Notes